KISS 10.10.10 DIET

Keeping it Super Simple 10 pounds, 10 days, 10 steps

Track Your Diet Success Diet Planner Food

Pyramid and Calorie Guide Included

KISS 10.10.10 Diet Plan

Lose 10 pounds in 10 days with 10 simple steps

Keeping It Super Simple (KISS) is the key to implementing and sticking to any weight loss plan. Here's how I lost 200 pounds in a year and a half.

1. *Commit and keep track with the enclosed journal.*
2. *Drink 64 ounces of water a day.*
3. *Eat 50% of Veggies and Fruit as your daily food intake.*
4. *Stick to consuming 1,000 calories a day.*
5. *Walk 20 Minutes 5 days a week.*
6. *Cut out Processed Foods. If it comes in a package do not eat it.*
7. *Meditate 15 minutes every night visualizing yourself thin.*
8. *Plan your meals for 10 days, prepare ahead to ensure success.*
9. *Take a Vitamin Supplement and a Probiotic in capsule form.*
10. *Take 10 deep breaths 3 times a day to aid in weight loss.*

Remember one person's food can be another person's poison. Listen to your body and if you eat something that makes you feel bad then don't eat it.

The enclosed eating guides are just as it says a guide and can be varied. As you can see for me I varied the guide to 50% of intake to be fresh raw fruits and veggies. Varying for me was perfect and can be for you too with my 10.10.10 rule, (lose 10 pounds in 10 days in 10 simple steps). No two people are alike and weightloss can and does vary from person to person. I can say when following my Kiss Plan you will lose weight.

I have been or tried just about every diet, diet pill, powders out there. My Kiss Diet is tried and true and will help you get to your goal weight one day at a time.

The content of this book is for general instruction only. Each person's physical, emotional, and spiritual condition is unique. The instruction in this book is not intended to replace or interrupt the reader's relationship with a physician or other professional. Please consult your doctor for matters pertaining to your specific health, diet and exercise.

Email receipt of purchse of this book to healthtidings@outlook.com and receive free digital handy lists grocery shopping such as all the hidden names in products, to check for MSG, other names of sugar, corn, toxins, chemicals, additives, flavoring agents and other lists.

Be sure to check out My story "Connecting the Dots" at www.healthtidings.com

The healthy eating pyramid

- Include breakfast in your daily plan
- Eat more often but smaller portions
- Avoid eating in fast foods
- Eat more vegetables and fruits

Eat sparingly:

- red meat, butter and salt
- refined grains: bread, white rice and pasta
- potatoes
- sweets and sugary drinks

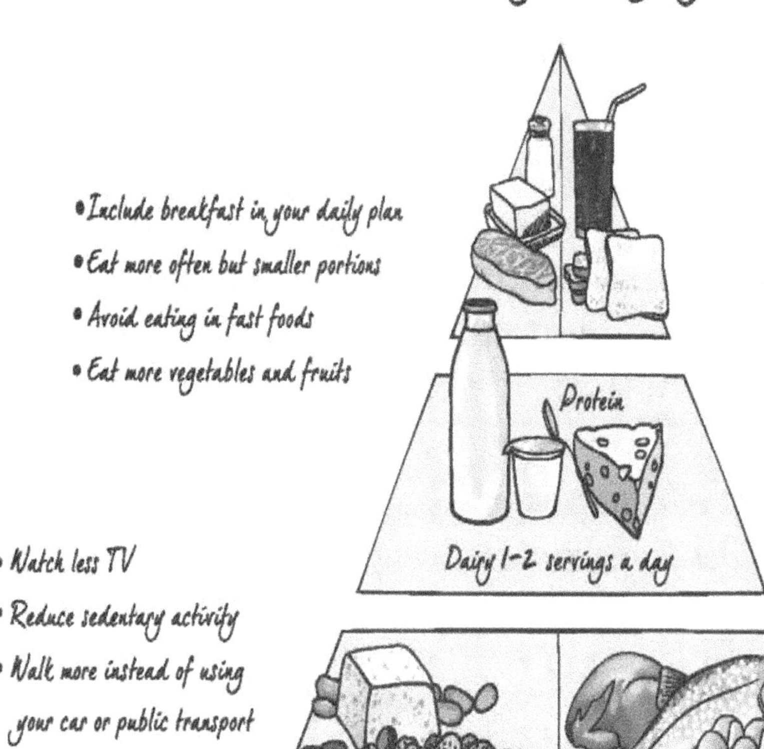

- Watch less TV
- Reduce sedentary activity
- Walk more instead of using your car or public transport
- Exercise more

Healthy fats and oils:
Olive, corn, soy, canola, sunflower and other vegetable oils.
Trans-free margarine.

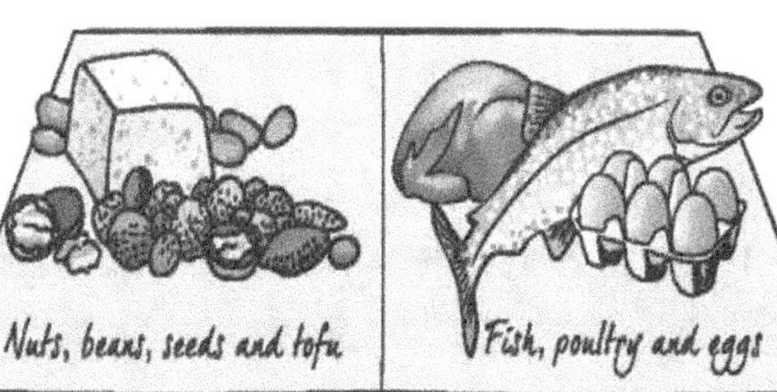

Whole grains:
Whole wheat pasta, brown rice, oats, etc.

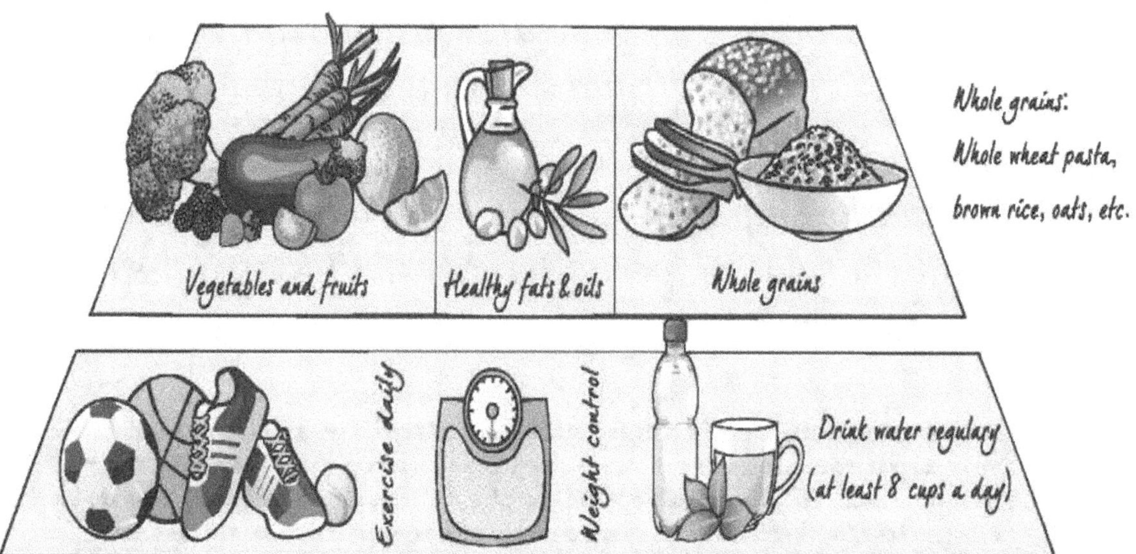

Drink 1-2 litres of liquid a day, preferably unsweetened.
Caffeinated beverages should be consumed in moderation only.

Calorie Counting Chart

List of Calories in Food

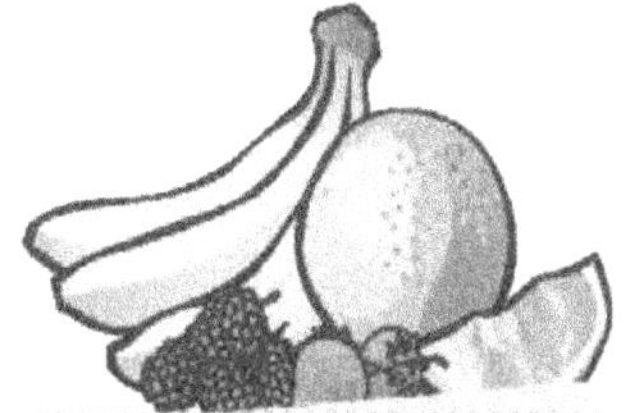

Calories in Fruits per 100 Grams

Apple	56 kcal	233 kJ
Avocado	190 kcal	795 kJ
Banana	95 kcal	397 kJ
Cherries	70 kcal	293 kJ
Dates	281 kcal	1175 kJ
Grapes Black	45 kcal	188 kJ
Guava	66 kcal	276 kJ
Kiwi Fruit	45 kcal	188 kJ
Mangoes	70 kcal	293 kJ
Orange	53 kcal	222 kJ
Orange juice 100ml	47 kcal	197 kJ
Papaya	32 kcal	134 kJ
Peach	50 kcal	209 kJ
Pears	51 kcal	214 kJ
Pineapple	46 kcal	193 kJ
Plums	56 kcal	234 kJ
Strawberries	77 kcal	322 kJ
Watermelon	26 kcal	109 kJ
Pomegranate	77 kcal	322 kJ
Watermelon	16 kcal	67 kJ

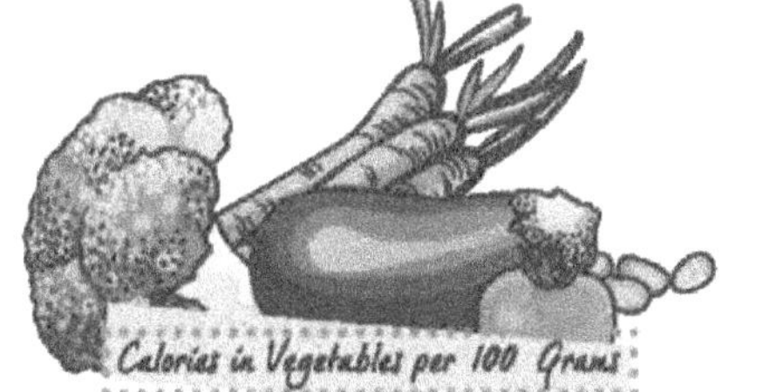

Calories in Vegetables per 100 Grams

Broccoli	25 kcal	105 kJ
Cabbage	45 kcal	188 kJ
Carrot	48 kcal	201 kJ
Cauliflower	30 kcal	126 kJ
Eggplant	27 kcal	113 kJ
French beans	26 kcal	109 kJ
Lettuce	21 kcal	88 kJ
Mushroom	18 kcal	75 kJ
Onion	50 kcal	209 kJ
Peas	93 kcal	389 kJ
Potato	97 kcal	406 kJ
Spinach 100g	26 kcal	109 kJ
Spinach 1 leaf	2 kcal	8 kJ
Spinach 1 bunch	78 kcal	326 kJ
Tomato	21 kcal	88 kJ
Tomato juice 100ml	22 kcal	92 kJ

Calories in Meat per 100 Grams

Bacon, average rashers	500 kcal	2090 kJ
Beef, average lean	275 kcal	1150 kJ
Lamb breast, roasted	398 kcal	1664 kJ
Lamb chops, grilled	368 kcal	1538 kJ
Lamb cutlets, grilled	375 kcal	1568 kJ
Lamb leg, roasted	270 kcal	1129 kJ
Lamb shoulder, roasted	320 kcal	1338 kJ
Pork belly rashers, grilled	400 kcal	1672 kJ
Pork chops, grilled	340 kcal	1421 kJ
Pork leg, roasted	290 kcal	1212 kJ
Pork trotters, boiled	290 kcal	1212 kJ
Veal fillet, roasted	240 kcal	1003 kJ
Chicken, average	140 kcal	585 kJ
Duck, roasted	330 kcal	1380 kJ
Goose, roasted	350 kcal	1463 kJ
Partridge, roasted	250 kcal	1045 kJ
Pheasant, roasted	250 kcal	1045 kJ
Pigeon, roasted	250 kcal	1045 kJ
Turkey, roasted	165 kcal	690 kJ
Hare	155 kcal	648 kJ
Rabbit	187 kcal	782 kJ
Venison	200 kcal	836 kJ

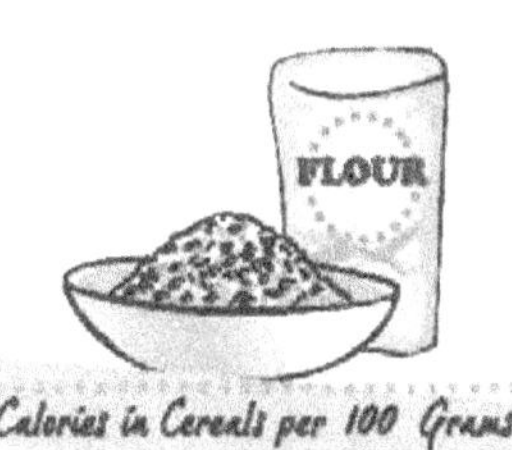

Calories in Cereals per 100 Grams

Bajra	360 kcal	1505 kJ
Maize flour	355 kcal	1484 kJ
Rice	325 kcal	1359 kJ
Wheat flour	341 kcal	1426 kJ

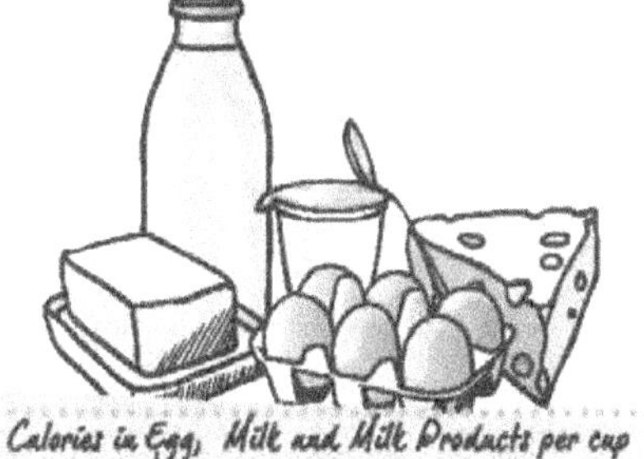

Calories in Egg, Milk and Milk Products per cup

Butter 100gms	750 kcal	3135 kJ
Buttermilk	19 kcal	80 kJ
Cheese	315 kcal	1317 kJ
Cream 100gms.	210 kcal	878 kJ
Eggs, Boiled	147 kcal	615 kJ
Ghee 100gms	910 kcal	3804 kJ
Milk Buffalo	115 kcal	481 kJ
Milk Cow	100 kcal	418 kJ
Milk Skimmed	45 kcal	188 kJ

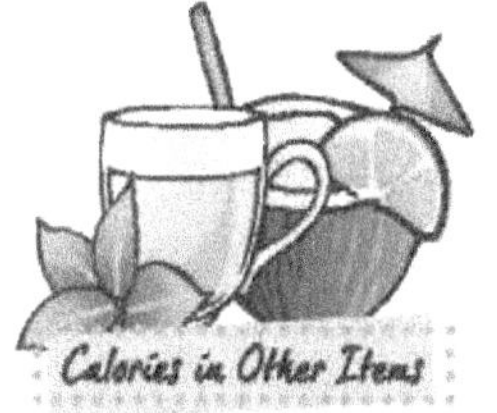

Calories in Other Items

Sugar 1 tbsp	48 kcal	200 kJ
Honey 1 tbsp	90 kcal	376 kJ
Coconut water 100 ml	25 kcal	105 kJ
Coffee	40 kcal	167 kJ
Tea	30 kcal	126 kJ

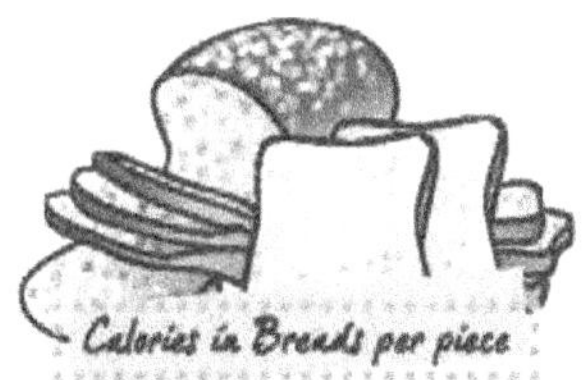

Calories in Breads per piece

1 medium chapati	119 kcal	478 kJ
1 slice white bread	60 kcal	251 kJ
1 paratha (no filling)	280 kcal	1171 kJ

1 kilojoule (kJ) = 1000 joules

1 kilocalorie = 1000 calories = 1 Calorie (1 Cal)

1 cal = 1 kcal = 4.18 kJ

PERSONAL GOALS

Start Date: End Date:

My Goals: ______________________________

____

____

My Plans: ______________________________

____

____

Daily Food Targets

calories

fat

carbs

fiber

protein

My Statistics

GOAL	RECORD ONE OR MORE	BEFORE	AFTER	NET +/-
	weight			
	cholesterol level			
	blood pressure			
	MEASUREMENTS:			
	chest			
	waist			
	hip			
	neck			
	upper arms			
	thighs			
	calves			

Before Pictures Here

After Pictures Here

DAY #: ___________

Meal 1	Portion Sizes		Fat	Calories	Carbs	Protein
TOTALS						
Satisfied after eating?						

Meal 2	Portion Sizes		Fat	Calories	Carbs	Protein
TOTALS						
Satisfied after eating?						

Notes

Meal 3	Portion Sizes	Fat	Calories	Carbs	Protein
TOTALS					
Satisfied after eating?					

Meal 4	Portion Sizes	Fat	Calories	Carbs	Protein
TOTALS					
Satisfied after eating?					

Meal 5	Portion Sizes	Fat	Calories	Carbs	Protein
TOTALS					
Satisfied after eating?					

DAY #: ___________

Meal 1	Portion Sizes	Fat	Calories	Carbs	Protein
TOTALS					
Satisfied after eating?					

Meal 2	Portion Sizes	Fat	Calories	Carbs	Protein
TOTALS					
Satisfied after eating?					

Notes

Meal 3	Portion Sizes	Fat	Calories	Carbs	Protein
TOTALS					
Satisfied after eating?					

Meal 4	Portion Sizes	Fat	Calories	Carbs	Protein
TOTALS					
Satisfied after eating?					

Meal 5	Portion Sizes	Fat	Calories	Carbs	Protein
TOTALS					
Satisfied after eating?					

DAY #:___________

Meal 1	Portion Sizes	Fat	Calories	Carbs	Protein
TOTALS					
Satisfied after eating?					

Meal 2	Portion Sizes	Fat	Calories	Carbs	Protein
TOTALS					
Satisfied after eating?					

Notes

Meal 3	Portion Sizes	Fat	Calories	Carbs	Protein
TOTALS					
Satisfied after eating?					

Meal 4	Portion Sizes	Fat	Calories	Carbs	Protein
TOTALS					
Satisfied after eating?					

Meal 5	Portion Sizes	Fat	Calories	Carbs	Protein
TOTALS					
Satisfied after eating?					

DAY #:___________

Meal 1	Portion Sizes	Fat	Calories	Carbs	Protein
TOTALS					
Satisfied after eating?					

Meal 2	Portion Sizes	Fat	Calories	Carbs	Protein
TOTALS					
Satisfied after eating?					

Notes

Meal 3	Portion Sizes	Fat	Calories	Carbs	Protein
TOTALS					
Satisfied after eating?					

Meal 4	Portion Sizes	Fat	Calories	Carbs	Protein
TOTALS					
Satisfied after eating?					

Meal 5	Portion Sizes	Fat	Calories	Carbs	Protein
TOTALS					
Satisfied after eating?					

DAY #:___________

Meal 1	Portion Sizes	Fat	Calories	Carbs	Protein
TOTALS					
Satisfied after eating?					

Meal 2	Portion Sizes	Fat	Calories	Carbs	Protein
TOTALS					
Satisfied after eating?					

Notes

Meal 3	Portion Sizes	Fat	Calories	Carbs	Protein
TOTALS					
Satisfied after eating?					

Meal 4	Portion Sizes	Fat	Calories	Carbs	Protein
TOTALS					
Satisfied after eating?					

Meal 5	Portion Sizes	Fat	Calories	Carbs	Protein
TOTALS					
Satisfied after eating?					

DAY #:___________

Meal 1	Portion Sizes	Fat	Calories	Carbs	Protein
TOTALS					
Satisfied after eating?					

Meal 2	Portion Sizes	Fat	Calories	Carbs	Protein
TOTALS					
Satisfied after eating?					

Notes

Meal 3	Portion Sizes	Fat	Calories	Carbs	Protein
TOTALS					
Satisfied after eating?					

Meal 4	Portion Sizes	Fat	Calories	Carbs	Protein
TOTALS					
Satisfied after eating?					

Meal 5	Portion Sizes	Fat	Calories	Carbs	Protein
TOTALS					
Satisfied after eating?					

DAY #:___________

Meal 1	Portion Sizes		Fat	Calories	Carbs	Protein
TOTALS						
Satisfied after eating?						

Meal 2	Portion Sizes		Fat	Calories	Carbs	Protein
TOTALS						
Satisfied after eating?						

Notes

Meal 3	Portion Sizes	Fat	Calories	Carbs	Protein
TOTALS					
Satisfied after eating?					

Meal 4	Portion Sizes	Fat	Calories	Carbs	Protein
TOTALS					
Satisfied after eating?					

Meal 5	Portion Sizes	Fat	Calories	Carbs	Protein
TOTALS					
Satisfied after eating?					

DAY #:___________

Meal 1	Portion Sizes		Fat	Calories	Carbs	Protein
TOTALS						
Satisfied after eating?						

Meal 2	Portion Sizes		Fat	Calories	Carbs	Protein
TOTALS						
Satisfied after eating?						

Notes

Meal 3	Portion Sizes	Fat	Calories	Carbs	Protein
TOTALS					
Satisfied after eating?					

Meal 4	Portion Sizes	Fat	Calories	Carbs	Protein
TOTALS					
Satisfied after eating?					

Meal 5	Portion Sizes	Fat	Calories	Carbs	Protein
TOTALS					
Satisfied after eating?					

DAY #:____________

Meal 1	Portion Sizes		Fat	Calories	Carbs	Protein
TOTALS						
Satisfied after eating?						

Meal 2	Portion Sizes		Fat	Calories	Carbs	Protein
TOTALS						
Satisfied after eating?						

Notes

Meal 3	Portion Sizes	Fat	Calories	Carbs	Protein
TOTALS					
Satisfied after eating?					

Meal 4	Portion Sizes	Fat	Calories	Carbs	Protein
TOTALS					
Satisfied after eating?					

Meal 5	Portion Sizes	Fat	Calories	Carbs	Protein
TOTALS					
Satisfied after eating?					

DAY #: ___________

Meal 1	Portion Sizes		Fat	Calories	Carbs	Protein
TOTALS						
Satisfied after eating?						

Meal 2	Portion Sizes		Fat	Calories	Carbs	Protein
TOTALS						
Satisfied after eating?						

Notes

Meal 3	Portion Sizes		Fat	Calories	Carbs	Protein
TOTALS						
Satisfied after eating?						

Meal 4	Portion Sizes		Fat	Calories	Carbs	Protein
TOTALS						
Satisfied after eating?						

Meal 5	Portion Sizes		Fat	Calories	Carbs	Protein
TOTALS						
Satisfied after eating?						

DAY #:____________

Meal 1	Portion Sizes		Fat	Calories	Carbs	Protein
TOTALS						
Satisfied after eating?						

Meal 2	Portion Sizes		Fat	Calories	Carbs	Protein
TOTALS						
Satisfied after eating?						

Notes

Meal 3	Portion Sizes	Fat	Calories	Carbs	Protein
TOTALS					
Satisfied after eating?					

Meal 4	Portion Sizes	Fat	Calories	Carbs	Protein
TOTALS					
Satisfied after eating?					

Meal 5	Portion Sizes	Fat	Calories	Carbs	Protein
TOTALS					
Satisfied after eating?					

DAY #:______________

Meal 1	Portion Sizes		Fat	Calories	Carbs	Protein
TOTALS						
Satisfied after eating?						

Meal 2	Portion Sizes		Fat	Calories	Carbs	Protein
TOTALS						
Satisfied after eating?						

Notes

Meal 3	Portion Sizes	Fat	Calories	Carbs	Protein
TOTALS					
Satisfied after eating?					

Meal 4	Portion Sizes	Fat	Calories	Carbs	Protein
TOTALS					
Satisfied after eating?					

Meal 5	Portion Sizes	Fat	Calories	Carbs	Protein
TOTALS					
Satisfied after eating?					

DAY #:___________

Meal 1	Portion Sizes		Fat	Calories	Carbs	Protein
TOTALS						
Satisfied after eating?						

Meal 2	Portion Sizes		Fat	Calories	Carbs	Protein
TOTALS						
Satisfied after eating?						

Notes

Meal 3	Portion Sizes	Fat	Calories	Carbs	Protein
TOTALS					
Satisfied after eating?					

Meal 4	Portion Sizes	Fat	Calories	Carbs	Protein
TOTALS					
Satisfied after eating?					

Meal 5	Portion Sizes	Fat	Calories	Carbs	Protein
TOTALS					
Satisfied after eating?					

DAY #:____________

Meal 1	Portion Sizes		Fat	Calories	Carbs	Protein
TOTALS						
Satisfied after eating?						

Meal 2	Portion Sizes		Fat	Calories	Carbs	Protein
TOTALS						
Satisfied after eating?						

Notes

Meal 3	Portion Sizes		Fat	Calories	Carbs	Protein
TOTALS						
Satisfied after eating?						

Meal 4	Portion Sizes		Fat	Calories	Carbs	Protein
TOTALS						
Satisfied after eating?						

Meal 5	Portion Sizes		Fat	Calories	Carbs	Protein
TOTALS						
Satisfied after eating?						

DAY #:___________

Meal 1	Portion Sizes		Fat	Calories	Carbs	Protein
TOTALS						
Satisfied after eating?						

Meal 2	Portion Sizes		Fat	Calories	Carbs	Protein
TOTALS						
Satisfied after eating?						

Notes

Meal 3	Portion Sizes	Fat	Calories	Carbs	Protein
TOTALS					
Satisfied after eating?					

Meal 4	Portion Sizes	Fat	Calories	Carbs	Protein
TOTALS					
Satisfied after eating?					

Meal 5	Portion Sizes	Fat	Calories	Carbs	Protein
TOTALS					
Satisfied after eating?					

DAY #:____________

Meal 1	Portion Sizes	Fat	Calories	Carbs	Protein
TOTALS					
Satisfied after eating?					

Meal 2	Portion Sizes	Fat	Calories	Carbs	Protein
TOTALS					
Satisfied after eating?					

Notes

Meal 3	Portion Sizes	Fat	Calories	Carbs	Protein
TOTALS					
Satisfied after eating?					

Meal 4	Portion Sizes	Fat	Calories	Carbs	Protein
TOTALS					
Satisfied after eating?					

Meal 5	Portion Sizes	Fat	Calories	Carbs	Protein
TOTALS					
Satisfied after eating?					

DAY #:____________

Meal 1	Portion Sizes	Fat	Calories	Carbs	Protein
TOTALS					
Satisfied after eating?					

Meal 2	Portion Sizes	Fat	Calories	Carbs	Protein
TOTALS					
Satisfied after eating?					

Notes

Meal 3	Portion Sizes	Fat	Calories	Carbs	Protein
TOTALS					
Satisfied after eating?					

Meal 4	Portion Sizes	Fat	Calories	Carbs	Protein
TOTALS					
Satisfied after eating?					

Meal 5	Portion Sizes	Fat	Calories	Carbs	Protein
TOTALS					
Satisfied after eating?					

DAY #:__________

Meal 1	Portion Sizes	Fat	Calories	Carbs	Protein
TOTALS					
Satisfied after eating?					

Meal 2	Portion Sizes	Fat	Calories	Carbs	Protein
TOTALS					
Satisfied after eating?					

Notes

Meal 3	Portion Sizes	Fat	Calories	Carbs	Protein
TOTALS					
Satisfied after eating?					

Meal 4	Portion Sizes	Fat	Calories	Carbs	Protein
TOTALS					
Satisfied after eating?					

Meal 5	Portion Sizes	Fat	Calories	Carbs	Protein
TOTALS					
Satisfied after eating?					

DAY #:____________

Meal 1	Portion Sizes	Fat	Calories	Carbs	Protein
TOTALS					
Satisfied after eating?					

Meal 2	Portion Sizes	Fat	Calories	Carbs	Protein
TOTALS					
Satisfied after eating?					

Notes

Meal 3	Portion Sizes	Fat	Calories	Carbs	Protein
TOTALS					
Satisfied after eating?					

Meal 4	Portion Sizes	Fat	Calories	Carbs	Protein
TOTALS					
Satisfied after eating?					

Meal 5	Portion Sizes	Fat	Calories	Carbs	Protein
TOTALS					
Satisfied after eating?					

DAY #:___________

Meal 1	Portion Sizes	Fat	Calories	Carbs	Protein
TOTALS					
Satisfied after eating?					

Meal 2	Portion Sizes	Fat	Calories	Carbs	Protein
TOTALS					
Satisfied after eating?					

Notes

Meal 3	Portion Sizes	Fat	Calories	Carbs	Protein
TOTALS					
Satisfied after eating?					

Meal 4	Portion Sizes	Fat	Calories	Carbs	Protein
TOTALS					
Satisfied after eating?					

Meal 5	Portion Sizes	Fat	Calories	Carbs	Protein
TOTALS					
Satisfied after eating?					

DAY #:___________

Meal 1	Portion Sizes		Fat	Calories	Carbs	Protein
TOTALS						
Satisfied after eating?						

Meal 2	Portion Sizes		Fat	Calories	Carbs	Protein
TOTALS						
Satisfied after eating?						

Notes

Meal 3	Portion Sizes	Fat	Calories	Carbs	Protein
TOTALS					
Satisfied after eating?					

Meal 4	Portion Sizes	Fat	Calories	Carbs	Protein
TOTALS					
Satisfied after eating?					

Meal 5	Portion Sizes	Fat	Calories	Carbs	Protein
TOTALS					
Satisfied after eating?					

DAY #:___________

Meal 1	Portion Sizes	Fat	Calories	Carbs	Protein
TOTALS					
Satisfied after eating?					

Meal 2	Portion Sizes	Fat	Calories	Carbs	Protein
TOTALS					
Satisfied after eating?					

Notes

Meal 3	Portion Sizes	Fat	Calories	Carbs	Protein
TOTALS					
Satisfied after eating?					

Meal 4	Portion Sizes	Fat	Calories	Carbs	Protein
TOTALS					
Satisfied after eating?					

Meal 5	Portion Sizes	Fat	Calories	Carbs	Protein
TOTALS					
Satisfied after eating?					

DAY #:___________

Meal 1	Portion Sizes	Fat	Calories	Carbs	Protein
TOTALS					
Satisfied after eating?					

Meal 2	Portion Sizes	Fat	Calories	Carbs	Protein
TOTALS					
Satisfied after eating?					

Notes

Meal 3	Portion Sizes	Fat	Calories	Carbs	Protein
TOTALS					
Satisfied after eating?					

Meal 4	Portion Sizes	Fat	Calories	Carbs	Protein
TOTALS					
Satisfied after eating?					

Meal 5	Portion Sizes	Fat	Calories	Carbs	Protein
TOTALS					
Satisfied after eating?					

DAY #:___________

Meal 1	Portion Sizes		Fat	Calories	Carbs	Protein
TOTALS						
Satisfied after eating?						

Meal 2	Portion Sizes		Fat	Calories	Carbs	Protein
TOTALS						
Satisfied after eating?						

Notes

Meal 3	Portion Sizes	Fat	Calories	Carbs	Protein
TOTALS					
Satisfied after eating?					

Meal 4	Portion Sizes	Fat	Calories	Carbs	Protein
TOTALS					
Satisfied after eating?					

Meal 5	Portion Sizes	Fat	Calories	Carbs	Protein
TOTALS					
Satisfied after eating?					

DAY #:___________

Meal 1	Portion Sizes		Fat	Calories	Carbs	Protein
TOTALS						
Satisfied after eating?						

Meal 2	Portion Sizes		Fat	Calories	Carbs	Protein
TOTALS						
Satisfied after eating?						

Notes

Meal 3	Portion Sizes	Fat	Calories	Carbs	Protein
TOTALS					
Satisfied after eating?					

Meal 4	Portion Sizes	Fat	Calories	Carbs	Protein
TOTALS					
Satisfied after eating?					

Meal 5	Portion Sizes	Fat	Calories	Carbs	Protein
TOTALS					
Satisfied after eating?					

DAY #:____________

Meal 1	Portion Sizes		Fat	Calories	Carbs	Protein
TOTALS						
Satisfied after eating?						

Meal 2	Portion Sizes		Fat	Calories	Carbs	Protein
TOTALS						
Satisfied after eating?						

Notes

Meal 3	Portion Sizes	Fat	Calories	Carbs	Protein
TOTALS					
Satisfied after eating?					

Meal 4	Portion Sizes	Fat	Calories	Carbs	Protein
TOTALS					
Satisfied after eating?					

Meal 5	Portion Sizes	Fat	Calories	Carbs	Protein
TOTALS					
Satisfied after eating?					

DAY #:__________

Meal 1	Portion Sizes	Fat	Calories	Carbs	Protein
TOTALS					
Satisfied after eating?					

Meal 2	Portion Sizes	Fat	Calories	Carbs	Protein
TOTALS					
Satisfied after eating?					

Notes

Meal 3	Portion Sizes	Fat	Calories	Carbs	Protein
TOTALS					
Satisfied after eating?					

Meal 4	Portion Sizes	Fat	Calories	Carbs	Protein
TOTALS					
Satisfied after eating?					

Meal 5	Portion Sizes	Fat	Calories	Carbs	Protein
TOTALS					
Satisfied after eating?					

DAY #:___________

Meal 1	Portion Sizes	Fat	Calories	Carbs	Protein
TOTALS					
Satisfied after eating?					

Meal 2	Portion Sizes	Fat	Calories	Carbs	Protein
TOTALS					
Satisfied after eating?					

Notes

Meal 3	Portion Sizes	Fat	Calories	Carbs	Protein
TOTALS					
Satisfied after eating?					

Meal 4	Portion Sizes	Fat	Calories	Carbs	Protein
TOTALS					
Satisfied after eating?					

Meal 5	Portion Sizes	Fat	Calories	Carbs	Protein
TOTALS					
Satisfied after eating?					

DAY #:____________

Meal 1	Portion Sizes	Fat	Calories	Carbs	Protein
TOTALS					
Satisfied after eating?					

Meal 2	Portion Sizes	Fat	Calories	Carbs	Protein
TOTALS					
Satisfied after eating?					

Notes

Meal 3	Portion Sizes	Fat	Calories	Carbs	Protein
TOTALS					
Satisfied after eating?					

Meal 4	Portion Sizes	Fat	Calories	Carbs	Protein
TOTALS					
Satisfied after eating?					

Meal 5	Portion Sizes	Fat	Calories	Carbs	Protein
TOTALS					
Satisfied after eating?					

DAY #:___________

Meal 1	Portion Sizes		Fat	Calories	Carbs	Protein
TOTALS						
Satisfied after eating?						

Meal 2	Portion Sizes		Fat	Calories	Carbs	Protein
TOTALS						
Satisfied after eating?						

Notes

Meal 3	Portion Sizes	Fat	Calories	Carbs	Protein
TOTALS					
Satisfied after eating?					

Meal 4	Portion Sizes	Fat	Calories	Carbs	Protein
TOTALS					
Satisfied after eating?					

Meal 5	Portion Sizes	Fat	Calories	Carbs	Protein
TOTALS					
Satisfied after eating?					

DAY #:____________

Meal 1	Portion Sizes		Fat	Calories	Carbs	Protein
TOTALS						
Satisfied after eating?						

Meal 2	Portion Sizes		Fat	Calories	Carbs	Protein
TOTALS						
Satisfied after eating?						

Notes

Meal 3	Portion Sizes		Fat	Calories	Carbs	Protein
TOTALS						
Satisfied after eating?						

Meal 4	Portion Sizes		Fat	Calories	Carbs	Protein
TOTALS						
Satisfied after eating?						

Meal 5	Portion Sizes		Fat	Calories	Carbs	Protein
TOTALS						
Satisfied after eating?						

DAY #:___________

Meal 1	Portion Sizes		Fat	Calories	Carbs	Protein
TOTALS						
Satisfied after eating?						

Meal 2	Portion Sizes		Fat	Calories	Carbs	Protein
TOTALS						
Satisfied after eating?						

Notes

Meal 3	Portion Sizes		Fat	Calories	Carbs	Protein
TOTALS						
Satisfied after eating?						

Meal 4	Portion Sizes		Fat	Calories	Carbs	Protein
TOTALS						
Satisfied after eating?						

Meal 5	Portion Sizes		Fat	Calories	Carbs	Protein
TOTALS						
Satisfied after eating?						

DAY #:___________

Meal 1	Portion Sizes	Fat	Calories	Carbs	Protein
TOTALS					
Satisfied after eating?					

Meal 2	Portion Sizes	Fat	Calories	Carbs	Protein
TOTALS					
Satisfied after eating?					

Notes

Meal 3	Portion Sizes	Fat	Calories	Carbs	Protein
TOTALS					
Satisfied after eating?					

Meal 4	Portion Sizes	Fat	Calories	Carbs	Protein
TOTALS					
Satisfied after eating?					

Meal 5	Portion Sizes	Fat	Calories	Carbs	Protein
TOTALS					
Satisfied after eating?					

DAY #:___________

Meal 1	Portion Sizes		Fat	Calories	Carbs	Protein
TOTALS						
Satisfied after eating?						

Meal 2	Portion Sizes		Fat	Calories	Carbs	Protein
TOTALS						
Satisfied after eating?						

Notes

Meal 3	Portion Sizes	Fat	Calories	Carbs	Protein
TOTALS					
Satisfied after eating?					

Meal 4	Portion Sizes	Fat	Calories	Carbs	Protein
TOTALS					
Satisfied after eating?					

Meal 5	Portion Sizes	Fat	Calories	Carbs	Protein
TOTALS					
Satisfied after eating?					

DAY #:_____________

Meal 1	Portion Sizes		Fat	Calories	Carbs	Protein
TOTALS						
Satisfied after eating?						

Meal 2	Portion Sizes		Fat	Calories	Carbs	Protein
TOTALS						
Satisfied after eating?						

Notes

Meal 3	Portion Sizes	Fat	Calories	Carbs	Protein
TOTALS					
Satisfied after eating?					

Meal 4	Portion Sizes	Fat	Calories	Carbs	Protein
TOTALS					
Satisfied after eating?					

Meal 5	Portion Sizes	Fat	Calories	Carbs	Protein
TOTALS					
Satisfied after eating?					

DAY #:____________

Meal 1	Portion Sizes	Fat	Calories	Carbs	Protein
TOTALS					
Satisfied after eating?					

Meal 2	Portion Sizes	Fat	Calories	Carbs	Protein
TOTALS					
Satisfied after eating?					

Notes

Meal 3	Portion Sizes		Fat	Calories	Carbs	Protein
TOTALS						
Satisfied after eating?						

Meal 4	Portion Sizes		Fat	Calories	Carbs	Protein
TOTALS						
Satisfied after eating?						

Meal 5	Portion Sizes		Fat	Calories	Carbs	Protein
TOTALS						
Satisfied after eating?						

DAY #:___________

Meal 1	Portion Sizes	Fat	Calories	Carbs	Protein
TOTALS					
Satisfied after eating?					

Meal 2	Portion Sizes	Fat	Calories	Carbs	Protein
TOTALS					
Satisfied after eating?					

Notes

Meal 3	Portion Sizes	Fat	Calories	Carbs	Protein
TOTALS					
Satisfied after eating?					

Meal 4	Portion Sizes	Fat	Calories	Carbs	Protein
TOTALS					
Satisfied after eating?					

Meal 5	Portion Sizes	Fat	Calories	Carbs	Protein
TOTALS					
Satisfied after eating?					

DAY #:___________

Meal 1	Portion Sizes	Fat	Calories	Carbs	Protein
TOTALS					
Satisfied after eating?					

Meal 2	Portion Sizes	Fat	Calories	Carbs	Protein
TOTALS					
Satisfied after eating?					

Notes

Meal 3	Portion Sizes	Fat	Calories	Carbs	Protein
TOTALS					
Satisfied after eating?					

Meal 4	Portion Sizes	Fat	Calories	Carbs	Protein
TOTALS					
Satisfied after eating?					

Meal 5	Portion Sizes	Fat	Calories	Carbs	Protein
TOTALS					
Satisfied after eating?					

DAY #:____________

Meal 1	Portion Sizes		Fat	Calories	Carbs	Protein
TOTALS						
Satisfied after eating?						

Meal 2	Portion Sizes		Fat	Calories	Carbs	Protein
TOTALS						
Satisfied after eating?						

Notes

Meal 3	Portion Sizes		Fat	Calories	Carbs	Protein
TOTALS						
Satisfied after eating?						

Meal 4	Portion Sizes		Fat	Calories	Carbs	Protein
TOTALS						
Satisfied after eating?						

Meal 5	Portion Sizes		Fat	Calories	Carbs	Protein
TOTALS						
Satisfied after eating?						

DAY #:____________

Meal 1	Portion Sizes	Fat	Calories	Carbs	Protein
TOTALS					
Satisfied after eating?					

Meal 2	Portion Sizes	Fat	Calories	Carbs	Protein
TOTALS					
Satisfied after eating?					

Notes

Meal 3	Portion Sizes	Fat	Calories	Carbs	Protein
TOTALS					
Satisfied after eating?					

Meal 4	Portion Sizes	Fat	Calories	Carbs	Protein
TOTALS					
Satisfied after eating?					

Meal 5	Portion Sizes	Fat	Calories	Carbs	Protein
TOTALS					
Satisfied after eating?					

DAY #:____________

Meal 1	Portion Sizes	Fat	Calories	Carbs	Protein
TOTALS					
Satisfied after eating?					

Meal 2	Portion Sizes	Fat	Calories	Carbs	Protein
TOTALS					
Satisfied after eating?					

Notes

Meal 3	Portion Sizes	Fat	Calories	Carbs	Protein
TOTALS					
Satisfied after eating?					

Meal 4	Portion Sizes	Fat	Calories	Carbs	Protein
TOTALS					
Satisfied after eating?					

Meal 5	Portion Sizes	Fat	Calories	Carbs	Protein
TOTALS					
Satisfied after eating?					

DAY #:____________

Meal 1	Portion Sizes	Fat	Calories	Carbs	Protein
TOTALS					
Satisfied after eating?					

Meal 2	Portion Sizes	Fat	Calories	Carbs	Protein
TOTALS					
Satisfied after eating?					

Notes

Meal 3	Portion Sizes	Fat	Calories	Carbs	Protein
TOTALS					
Satisfied after eating?					

Meal 4	Portion Sizes	Fat	Calories	Carbs	Protein
TOTALS					
Satisfied after eating?					

Meal 5	Portion Sizes	Fat	Calories	Carbs	Protein
TOTALS					
Satisfied after eating?					

DAY #:____________

Meal 1	Portion Sizes		Fat	Calories	Carbs	Protein
TOTALS						
Satisfied after eating?						

Meal 2	Portion Sizes		Fat	Calories	Carbs	Protein
TOTALS						
Satisfied after eating?						

Notes

Meal 3	Portion Sizes	Fat	Calories	Carbs	Protein
TOTALS					
Satisfied after eating?					

Meal 4	Portion Sizes	Fat	Calories	Carbs	Protein
TOTALS					
Satisfied after eating?					

Meal 5	Portion Sizes	Fat	Calories	Carbs	Protein
TOTALS					
Satisfied after eating?					

DAY #:____________

Meal 1	Portion Sizes		Fat	Calories	Carbs	Protein
TOTALS						
Satisfied after eating?						

Meal 2	Portion Sizes		Fat	Calories	Carbs	Protein
TOTALS						
Satisfied after eating?						

Notes

Meal 3	Portion Sizes	Fat	Calories	Carbs	Protein
TOTALS					
Satisfied after eating?					

Meal 4	Portion Sizes	Fat	Calories	Carbs	Protein
TOTALS					
Satisfied after eating?					

Meal 5	Portion Sizes	Fat	Calories	Carbs	Protein
TOTALS					
Satisfied after eating?					

DAY #:____________

Meal 1	Portion Sizes		Fat	Calories	Carbs	Protein
TOTALS						
Satisfied after eating?						

Meal 2	Portion Sizes		Fat	Calories	Carbs	Protein
TOTALS						
Satisfied after eating?						

Notes

Meal 3	Portion Sizes	Fat	Calories	Carbs	Protein
TOTALS					
Satisfied after eating?					

Meal 4	Portion Sizes	Fat	Calories	Carbs	Protein
TOTALS					
Satisfied after eating?					

Meal 5	Portion Sizes	Fat	Calories	Carbs	Protein
TOTALS					
Satisfied after eating?					

DAY #:____________

Meal 1	Portion Sizes	Fat	Calories	Carbs	Protein
TOTALS					
Satisfied after eating?					

Meal 2	Portion Sizes	Fat	Calories	Carbs	Protein
TOTALS					
Satisfied after eating?					

Notes

Meal 3	Portion Sizes	Fat	Calories	Carbs	Protein
TOTALS					
Satisfied after eating?					

Meal 4	Portion Sizes	Fat	Calories	Carbs	Protein
TOTALS					
Satisfied after eating?					

Meal 5	Portion Sizes	Fat	Calories	Carbs	Protein
TOTALS					
Satisfied after eating?					

DAY #:___________

Meal 1	Portion Sizes	Fat	Calories	Carbs	Protein
TOTALS					
Satisfied after eating?					

Meal 2	Portion Sizes	Fat	Calories	Carbs	Protein
TOTALS					
Satisfied after eating?					

Notes

Meal 3	Portion Sizes	Fat	Calories	Carbs	Protein
TOTALS					
Satisfied after eating?					

Meal 4	Portion Sizes	Fat	Calories	Carbs	Protein
TOTALS					
Satisfied after eating?					

Meal 5	Portion Sizes	Fat	Calories	Carbs	Protein
TOTALS					
Satisfied after eating?					

DAY #:___________

Meal 1	Portion Sizes	Fat	Calories	Carbs	Protein
TOTALS					
Satisfied after eating?					

Meal 2	Portion Sizes	Fat	Calories	Carbs	Protein
TOTALS					
Satisfied after eating?					

Notes

Meal 3	Portion Sizes	Fat	Calories	Carbs	Protein
TOTALS					
Satisfied after eating?					

Meal 4	Portion Sizes	Fat	Calories	Carbs	Protein
TOTALS					
Satisfied after eating?					

Meal 5	Portion Sizes	Fat	Calories	Carbs	Protein
TOTALS					
Satisfied after eating?					

DAY #:____________

Meal 1	Portion Sizes	Fat	Calories	Carbs	Protein
TOTALS					
Satisfied after eating?					

Meal 2	Portion Sizes	Fat	Calories	Carbs	Protein
TOTALS					
Satisfied after eating?					

Notes

Meal 3	Portion Sizes	Fat	Calories	Carbs	Protein
TOTALS					
Satisfied after eating?					

Meal 4	Portion Sizes	Fat	Calories	Carbs	Protein
TOTALS					
Satisfied after eating?					

Meal 5	Portion Sizes	Fat	Calories	Carbs	Protein
TOTALS					
Satisfied after eating?					

DAY #:___________

Meal 1	Portion Sizes		Fat	Calories	Carbs	Protein
TOTALS						
Satisfied after eating?						

Meal 2	Portion Sizes		Fat	Calories	Carbs	Protein
TOTALS						
Satisfied after eating?						

Notes

Meal 3	Portion Sizes	Fat	Calories	Carbs	Protein
TOTALS					
Satisfied after eating?					

Meal 4	Portion Sizes	Fat	Calories	Carbs	Protein
TOTALS					
Satisfied after eating?					

Meal 5	Portion Sizes	Fat	Calories	Carbs	Protein
TOTALS					
Satisfied after eating?					

DAY #:____________

Meal 1	Portion Sizes	Fat	Calories	Carbs	Protein
TOTALS					
Satisfied after eating?					

Meal 2	Portion Sizes	Fat	Calories	Carbs	Protein
TOTALS					
Satisfied after eating?					

Notes

Meal 3	Portion Sizes	Fat	Calories	Carbs	Protein
TOTALS					
Satisfied after eating?					

Meal 4	Portion Sizes	Fat	Calories	Carbs	Protein
TOTALS					
Satisfied after eating?					

Meal 5	Portion Sizes	Fat	Calories	Carbs	Protein
TOTALS					
Satisfied after eating?					

DAY #:___________

Meal 1	Portion Sizes	Fat	Calories	Carbs	Protein
TOTALS					
Satisfied after eating?					

Meal 2	Portion Sizes	Fat	Calories	Carbs	Protein
TOTALS					
Satisfied after eating?					

Notes

Meal 3	Portion Sizes		Fat	Calories	Carbs	Protein
TOTALS						
Satisfied after eating?						

Meal 4	Portion Sizes		Fat	Calories	Carbs	Protein
TOTALS						
Satisfied after eating?						

Meal 5	Portion Sizes		Fat	Calories	Carbs	Protein
TOTALS						
Satisfied after eating?						

DAY #:____________

Meal 1	Portion Sizes		Fat	Calories	Carbs	Protein
TOTALS						
Satisfied after eating?						

Meal 2	Portion Sizes		Fat	Calories	Carbs	Protein
TOTALS						
Satisfied after eating?						

Notes

Meal 3	Portion Sizes		Fat	Calories	Carbs	Protein
TOTALS						
Satisfied after eating?						

Meal 4	Portion Sizes		Fat	Calories	Carbs	Protein
TOTALS						
Satisfied after eating?						

Meal 5	Portion Sizes		Fat	Calories	Carbs	Protein
TOTALS						
Satisfied after eating?						

DAY #:____________

Meal 1	Portion Sizes	Fat	Calories	Carbs	Protein
TOTALS					
Satisfied after eating?					

Meal 2	Portion Sizes	Fat	Calories	Carbs	Protein
TOTALS					
Satisfied after eating?					

Notes

Meal 3	Portion Sizes	Fat	Calories	Carbs	Protein
TOTALS					
Satisfied after eating?					

Meal 4	Portion Sizes	Fat	Calories	Carbs	Protein
TOTALS					
Satisfied after eating?					

Meal 5	Portion Sizes	Fat	Calories	Carbs	Protein
TOTALS					
Satisfied after eating?					

DAY #:___________

Meal 1	Portion Sizes	Fat	Calories	Carbs	Protein
TOTALS					
Satisfied after eating?					

Meal 2	Portion Sizes	Fat	Calories	Carbs	Protein
TOTALS					
Satisfied after eating?					

Notes

Meal 3	Portion Sizes	Fat	Calories	Carbs	Protein
TOTALS					
Satisfied after eating?					

Meal 4	Portion Sizes	Fat	Calories	Carbs	Protein
TOTALS					
Satisfied after eating?					

Meal 5	Portion Sizes	Fat	Calories	Carbs	Protein
TOTALS					
Satisfied after eating?					

DAY #:___________

Meal 1	Portion Sizes	Fat	Calories	Carbs	Protein
TOTALS					
Satisfied after eating?					

Meal 2	Portion Sizes	Fat	Calories	Carbs	Protein
TOTALS					
Satisfied after eating?					

Notes

Meal 3	Portion Sizes	Fat	Calories	Carbs	Protein
TOTALS					
Satisfied after eating?					

Meal 4	Portion Sizes	Fat	Calories	Carbs	Protein
TOTALS					
Satisfied after eating?					

Meal 5	Portion Sizes	Fat	Calories	Carbs	Protein
TOTALS					
Satisfied after eating?					

DAY #:___________

Meal 1	Portion Sizes		Fat	Calories	Carbs	Protein
TOTALS						
Satisfied after eating?						

Meal 2	Portion Sizes		Fat	Calories	Carbs	Protein
TOTALS						
Satisfied after eating?						

Notes

Meal 3	Portion Sizes	Fat	Calories	Carbs	Protein
TOTALS					
Satisfied after eating?					

Meal 4	Portion Sizes	Fat	Calories	Carbs	Protein
TOTALS					
Satisfied after eating?					

Meal 5	Portion Sizes	Fat	Calories	Carbs	Protein
TOTALS					
Satisfied after eating?					

DAY #:___________

Meal 1	Portion Sizes	Fat	Calories	Carbs	Protein
TOTALS					
Satisfied after eating?					

Meal 2	Portion Sizes	Fat	Calories	Carbs	Protein
TOTALS					
Satisfied after eating?					

Notes

Meal 3	Portion Sizes	Fat	Calories	Carbs	Protein
TOTALS					
Satisfied after eating?					

Meal 4	Portion Sizes	Fat	Calories	Carbs	Protein
TOTALS					
Satisfied after eating?					

Meal 5	Portion Sizes	Fat	Calories	Carbs	Protein
TOTALS					
Satisfied after eating?					

DAY #:____________

Meal 1	Portion Sizes	Fat	Calories	Carbs	Protein
TOTALS					
Satisfied after eating?					

Meal 2	Portion Sizes	Fat	Calories	Carbs	Protein
TOTALS					
Satisfied after eating?					

Notes

Meal 3	Portion Sizes	Fat	Calories	Carbs	Protein
TOTALS					
Satisfied after eating?					

Meal 4	Portion Sizes	Fat	Calories	Carbs	Protein
TOTALS					
Satisfied after eating?					

Meal 5	Portion Sizes	Fat	Calories	Carbs	Protein
TOTALS					
Satisfied after eating?					

DAY #:___________

Meal 1	Portion Sizes	Fat	Calories	Carbs	Protein
TOTALS					
Satisfied after eating?					

Meal 2	Portion Sizes	Fat	Calories	Carbs	Protein
TOTALS					
Satisfied after eating?					

Notes

Meal 3	Portion Sizes	Fat	Calories	Carbs	Protein
TOTALS					
Satisfied after eating?					

Meal 4	Portion Sizes	Fat	Calories	Carbs	Protein
TOTALS					
Satisfied after eating?					

Meal 5	Portion Sizes	Fat	Calories	Carbs	Protein
TOTALS					
Satisfied after eating?					

DAY #:____________

Meal 1	Portion Sizes		Fat	Calories	Carbs	Protein
TOTALS						
Satisfied after eating?						

Meal 2	Portion Sizes		Fat	Calories	Carbs	Protein
TOTALS						
Satisfied after eating?						

Notes

Meal 3	Portion Sizes		Fat	Calories	Carbs	Protein
TOTALS						
Satisfied after eating?						

Meal 4	Portion Sizes		Fat	Calories	Carbs	Protein
TOTALS						
Satisfied after eating?						

Meal 5	Portion Sizes		Fat	Calories	Carbs	Protein
TOTALS						
Satisfied after eating?						

DAY #:___________

Meal 1	Portion Sizes		Fat	Calories	Carbs	Protein
TOTALS						
Satisfied after eating?						

Meal 2	Portion Sizes		Fat	Calories	Carbs	Protein
TOTALS						
Satisfied after eating?						

Notes

Meal 3	Portion Sizes	Fat	Calories	Carbs	Protein
TOTALS					
Satisfied after eating?					

Meal 4	Portion Sizes	Fat	Calories	Carbs	Protein
TOTALS					
Satisfied after eating?					

Meal 5	Portion Sizes	Fat	Calories	Carbs	Protein
TOTALS					
Satisfied after eating?					

DAY #:___________

Meal 1	Portion Sizes	Fat	Calories	Carbs	Protein
TOTALS					
Satisfied after eating?					

Meal 2	Portion Sizes	Fat	Calories	Carbs	Protein
TOTALS					
Satisfied after eating?					

Notes

Meal 3	Portion Sizes		Fat	Calories	Carbs	Protein
TOTALS						
Satisfied after eating?						

Meal 4	Portion Sizes		Fat	Calories	Carbs	Protein
TOTALS						
Satisfied after eating?						

Meal 5	Portion Sizes		Fat	Calories	Carbs	Protein
TOTALS						
Satisfied after eating?						

DAY #:____________

Meal 1	Portion Sizes	Fat	Calories	Carbs	Protein
TOTALS					
Satisfied after eating?					

Meal 2	Portion Sizes	Fat	Calories	Carbs	Protein
TOTALS					
Satisfied after eating?					

Notes

Meal 3	Portion Sizes	Fat	Calories	Carbs	Protein
TOTALS					
Satisfied after eating?					

Meal 4	Portion Sizes	Fat	Calories	Carbs	Protein
TOTALS					
Satisfied after eating?					

Meal 5	Portion Sizes	Fat	Calories	Carbs	Protein
TOTALS					
Satisfied after eating?					

DAY #:____________

Meal 1	Portion Sizes		Fat	Calories	Carbs	Protein
TOTALS						
Satisfied after eating?						

Meal 2	Portion Sizes		Fat	Calories	Carbs	Protein
TOTALS						
Satisfied after eating?						

Notes

Meal 3	Portion Sizes	Fat	Calories	Carbs	Protein
TOTALS					
Satisfied after eating?					

Meal 4	Portion Sizes	Fat	Calories	Carbs	Protein
TOTALS					
Satisfied after eating?					

Meal 5	Portion Sizes	Fat	Calories	Carbs	Protein
TOTALS					
Satisfied after eating?					

DAY #:___________

Meal 1	Portion Sizes	Fat	Calories	Carbs	Protein
TOTALS					
Satisfied after eating?					

Meal 2	Portion Sizes	Fat	Calories	Carbs	Protein
TOTALS					
Satisfied after eating?					

Notes

Meal 3	Portion Sizes	Fat	Calories	Carbs	Protein
TOTALS					
Satisfied after eating?					

Meal 4	Portion Sizes	Fat	Calories	Carbs	Protein
TOTALS					
Satisfied after eating?					

Meal 5	Portion Sizes	Fat	Calories	Carbs	Protein
TOTALS					
Satisfied after eating?					

DAY #:____________

Meal 1	Portion Sizes	Fat	Calories	Carbs	Protein
TOTALS					
Satisfied after eating?					

Meal 2	Portion Sizes	Fat	Calories	Carbs	Protein
TOTALS					
Satisfied after eating?					

Notes

Meal 3	Portion Sizes		Fat	Calories	Carbs	Protein
TOTALS						
Satisfied after eating?						

Meal 4	Portion Sizes		Fat	Calories	Carbs	Protein
TOTALS						
Satisfied after eating?						

Meal 5	Portion Sizes		Fat	Calories	Carbs	Protein
TOTALS						
Satisfied after eating?						

DAY #:___________

Meal 1	Portion Sizes	Fat	Calories	Carbs	Protein
TOTALS					
Satisfied after eating?					

Meal 2	Portion Sizes	Fat	Calories	Carbs	Protein
TOTALS					
Satisfied after eating?					

Notes

Meal 3	Portion Sizes	Fat	Calories	Carbs	Protein
TOTALS					
Satisfied after eating?					

Meal 4	Portion Sizes	Fat	Calories	Carbs	Protein
TOTALS					
Satisfied after eating?					

Meal 5	Portion Sizes	Fat	Calories	Carbs	Protein
TOTALS					
Satisfied after eating?					

DAY #:____________

Meal 1	Portion Sizes	Fat	Calories	Carbs	Protein
TOTALS					
Satisfied after eating?					

Meal 2	Portion Sizes	Fat	Calories	Carbs	Protein
TOTALS					
Satisfied after eating?					

Notes

Meal 3	Portion Sizes	Fat	Calories	Carbs	Protein
TOTALS					
Satisfied after eating?					

Meal 4	Portion Sizes	Fat	Calories	Carbs	Protein
TOTALS					
Satisfied after eating?					

Meal 5	Portion Sizes	Fat	Calories	Carbs	Protein
TOTALS					
Satisfied after eating?					

DAY #: ____________

Meal 1	Portion Sizes	Fat	Calories	Carbs	Protein
TOTALS					
Satisfied after eating?					

Meal 2	Portion Sizes	Fat	Calories	Carbs	Protein
TOTALS					
Satisfied after eating?					

Notes

Meal 3	Portion Sizes	Fat	Calories	Carbs	Protein
TOTALS					
Satisfied after eating?					

Meal 4	Portion Sizes	Fat	Calories	Carbs	Protein
TOTALS					
Satisfied after eating?					

Meal 5	Portion Sizes	Fat	Calories	Carbs	Protein
TOTALS					
Satisfied after eating?					

DAY #:____________

Meal 1	Portion Sizes	Fat	Calories	Carbs	Protein
TOTALS					
Satisfied after eating?					

Meal 2	Portion Sizes	Fat	Calories	Carbs	Protein
TOTALS					
Satisfied after eating?					

Notes

Meal 3	Portion Sizes	Fat	Calories	Carbs	Protein
TOTALS					
Satisfied after eating?					

Meal 4	Portion Sizes	Fat	Calories	Carbs	Protein
TOTALS					
Satisfied after eating?					

Meal 5	Portion Sizes	Fat	Calories	Carbs	Protein
TOTALS					
Satisfied after eating?					

DAY #:___________

Meal 1	Portion Sizes	Fat	Calories	Carbs	Protein
TOTALS					
Satisfied after eating?					

Meal 2	Portion Sizes	Fat	Calories	Carbs	Protein
TOTALS					
Satisfied after eating?					

Notes

Meal 3	Portion Sizes	Fat	Calories	Carbs	Protein
TOTALS					
Satisfied after eating?					

Meal 4	Portion Sizes	Fat	Calories	Carbs	Protein
TOTALS					
Satisfied after eating?					

Meal 5	Portion Sizes	Fat	Calories	Carbs	Protein
TOTALS					
Satisfied after eating?					

DAY #:____________

Meal 1	Portion Sizes	Fat	Calories	Carbs	Protein
TOTALS					
Satisfied after eating?					

Meal 2	Portion Sizes	Fat	Calories	Carbs	Protein
TOTALS					
Satisfied after eating?					

Notes

Meal 3	Portion Sizes	Fat	Calories	Carbs	Protein
TOTALS					
Satisfied after eating?					

Meal 4	Portion Sizes	Fat	Calories	Carbs	Protein
TOTALS					
Satisfied after eating?					

Meal 5	Portion Sizes	Fat	Calories	Carbs	Protein
TOTALS					
Satisfied after eating?					

DAY #:__________

Meal 1	Portion Sizes	Fat	Calories	Carbs	Protein
TOTALS					
Satisfied after eating?					

Meal 2	Portion Sizes	Fat	Calories	Carbs	Protein
TOTALS					
Satisfied after eating?					

Notes

Meal 3	Portion Sizes	Fat	Calories	Carbs	Protein
TOTALS					
Satisfied after eating?					

Meal 4	Portion Sizes	Fat	Calories	Carbs	Protein
TOTALS					
Satisfied after eating?					

Meal 5	Portion Sizes	Fat	Calories	Carbs	Protein
TOTALS					
Satisfied after eating?					

DAY #:__________

Meal 1	Portion Sizes		Fat	Calories	Carbs	Protein
TOTALS						
Satisfied after eating?						

Meal 2	Portion Sizes		Fat	Calories	Carbs	Protein
TOTALS						
Satisfied after eating?						

Notes

Meal 3	Portion Sizes		Fat	Calories	Carbs	Protein
TOTALS						
Satisfied after eating?						

Meal 4	Portion Sizes		Fat	Calories	Carbs	Protein
TOTALS						
Satisfied after eating?						

Meal 5	Portion Sizes		Fat	Calories	Carbs	Protein
TOTALS						
Satisfied after eating?						

DAY #:___________

Meal 1	Portion Sizes		Fat	Calories	Carbs	Protein
TOTALS						
Satisfied after eating?						

Meal 2	Portion Sizes		Fat	Calories	Carbs	Protein
TOTALS						
Satisfied after eating?						

Notes

Meal 3	Portion Sizes	Fat	Calories	Carbs	Protein
TOTALS					
Satisfied after eating?					

Meal 4	Portion Sizes	Fat	Calories	Carbs	Protein
TOTALS					
Satisfied after eating?					

Meal 5	Portion Sizes	Fat	Calories	Carbs	Protein
TOTALS					
Satisfied after eating?					

DAY #:___________

Meal 1	Portion Sizes	Fat	Calories	Carbs	Protein
TOTALS					
Satisfied after eating?					

Meal 2	Portion Sizes	Fat	Calories	Carbs	Protein
TOTALS					
Satisfied after eating?					

Notes

Meal 3	Portion Sizes	Fat	Calories	Carbs	Protein
TOTALS					
Satisfied after eating?					

Meal 4	Portion Sizes	Fat	Calories	Carbs	Protein
TOTALS					
Satisfied after eating?					

Meal 5	Portion Sizes	Fat	Calories	Carbs	Protein
TOTALS					
Satisfied after eating?					

DAY #:___________

Meal 1	Portion Sizes	Fat	Calories	Carbs	Protein
TOTALS					
Satisfied after eating?					

Meal 2	Portion Sizes	Fat	Calories	Carbs	Protein
TOTALS					
Satisfied after eating?					

Notes

Meal 3	Portion Sizes	Fat	Calories	Carbs	Protein
TOTALS					
Satisfied after eating?					

Meal 4	Portion Sizes	Fat	Calories	Carbs	Protein
TOTALS					
Satisfied after eating?					

Meal 5	Portion Sizes	Fat	Calories	Carbs	Protein
TOTALS					
Satisfied after eating?					

DAY #:__________

Meal 1	Portion Sizes	Fat	Calories	Carbs	Protein
TOTALS					
Satisfied after eating?					

Meal 2	Portion Sizes	Fat	Calories	Carbs	Protein
TOTALS					
Satisfied after eating?					

Notes

Meal 3	Portion Sizes	Fat	Calories	Carbs	Protein
TOTALS					
Satisfied after eating?					

Meal 4	Portion Sizes	Fat	Calories	Carbs	Protein
TOTALS					
Satisfied after eating?					

Meal 5	Portion Sizes	Fat	Calories	Carbs	Protein
TOTALS					
Satisfied after eating?					

DAY #:____________

Meal 1	Portion Sizes	Fat	Calories	Carbs	Protein
TOTALS					
Satisfied after eating?					

Meal 2	Portion Sizes	Fat	Calories	Carbs	Protein
TOTALS					
Satisfied after eating?					

Notes

Meal 3	Portion Sizes	Fat	Calories	Carbs	Protein
TOTALS					
Satisfied after eating?					

Meal 4	Portion Sizes	Fat	Calories	Carbs	Protein
TOTALS					
Satisfied after eating?					

Meal 5	Portion Sizes	Fat	Calories	Carbs	Protein
TOTALS					
Satisfied after eating?					

DAY #:___________

Meal 1	Portion Sizes	Fat	Calories	Carbs	Protein
TOTALS					
Satisfied after eating?					

Meal 2	Portion Sizes	Fat	Calories	Carbs	Protein
TOTALS					
Satisfied after eating?					

Notes

Meal 3	Portion Sizes	Fat	Calories	Carbs	Protein
TOTALS					
Satisfied after eating?					

Meal 4	Portion Sizes	Fat	Calories	Carbs	Protein
TOTALS					
Satisfied after eating?					

Meal 5	Portion Sizes	Fat	Calories	Carbs	Protein
TOTALS					
Satisfied after eating?					

DAY #:___________

Meal 1	Portion Sizes		Fat	Calories	Carbs	Protein
TOTALS						
Satisfied after eating?						

Meal 2	Portion Sizes		Fat	Calories	Carbs	Protein
TOTALS						
Satisfied after eating?						

Notes

Meal 3	Portion Sizes	Fat	Calories	Carbs	Protein
TOTALS					
Satisfied after eating?					

Meal 4	Portion Sizes	Fat	Calories	Carbs	Protein
TOTALS					
Satisfied after eating?					

Meal 5	Portion Sizes	Fat	Calories	Carbs	Protein
TOTALS					
Satisfied after eating?					

DAY #:____________

Meal 1	Portion Sizes		Fat	Calories	Carbs	Protein
TOTALS						
Satisfied after eating?						

Meal 2	Portion Sizes		Fat	Calories	Carbs	Protein
TOTALS						
Satisfied after eating?						

Notes

Meal 3	Portion Sizes	Fat	Calories	Carbs	Protein
TOTALS					
Satisfied after eating?					

Meal 4	Portion Sizes	Fat	Calories	Carbs	Protein
TOTALS					
Satisfied after eating?					

Meal 5	Portion Sizes	Fat	Calories	Carbs	Protein
TOTALS					
Satisfied after eating?					

DAY #:___________

Meal 1	Portion Sizes		Fat	Calories	Carbs	Protein
TOTALS						
Satisfied after eating?						

Meal 2	Portion Sizes		Fat	Calories	Carbs	Protein
TOTALS						
Satisfied after eating?						

Notes

Meal 3	Portion Sizes	Fat	Calories	Carbs	Protein
TOTALS					
Satisfied after eating?					

Meal 4	Portion Sizes	Fat	Calories	Carbs	Protein
TOTALS					
Satisfied after eating?					

Meal 5	Portion Sizes	Fat	Calories	Carbs	Protein
TOTALS					
Satisfied after eating?					

DAY #:____________

Meal 1	Portion Sizes	Fat	Calories	Carbs	Protein
TOTALS					
Satisfied after eating?					

Meal 2	Portion Sizes	Fat	Calories	Carbs	Protein
TOTALS					
Satisfied after eating?					

Notes

Meal 3	Portion Sizes	Fat	Calories	Carbs	Protein
TOTALS					
Satisfied after eating?					

Meal 4	Portion Sizes	Fat	Calories	Carbs	Protein
TOTALS					
Satisfied after eating?					

Meal 5	Portion Sizes	Fat	Calories	Carbs	Protein
TOTALS					
Satisfied after eating?					

DAY #:____________

Meal 1	Portion Sizes	Fat	Calories	Carbs	Protein
TOTALS					
Satisfied after eating?					

Meal 2	Portion Sizes	Fat	Calories	Carbs	Protein
TOTALS					
Satisfied after eating?					

Notes

Meal 3	Portion Sizes	Fat	Calories	Carbs	Protein
TOTALS					
Satisfied after eating?					

Meal 4	Portion Sizes	Fat	Calories	Carbs	Protein
TOTALS					
Satisfied after eating?					

Meal 5	Portion Sizes	Fat	Calories	Carbs	Protein
TOTALS					
Satisfied after eating?					

DAY #:____________

Meal 1	Portion Sizes	Fat	Calories	Carbs	Protein
TOTALS					
Satisfied after eating?					

Meal 2	Portion Sizes	Fat	Calories	Carbs	Protein
TOTALS					
Satisfied after eating?					

Notes

Meal 3	Portion Sizes	Fat	Calories	Carbs	Protein
TOTALS					
Satisfied after eating?					

Meal 4	Portion Sizes	Fat	Calories	Carbs	Protein
TOTALS					
Satisfied after eating?					

Meal 5	Portion Sizes	Fat	Calories	Carbs	Protein
TOTALS					
Satisfied after eating?					

DAY #:____________

Meal 1	Portion Sizes	Fat	Calories	Carbs	Protein
TOTALS					
Satisfied after eating?					

Meal 2	Portion Sizes	Fat	Calories	Carbs	Protein
TOTALS					
Satisfied after eating?					

Notes

Meal 3	Portion Sizes	Fat	Calories	Carbs	Protein
TOTALS					
Satisfied after eating?					

Meal 4	Portion Sizes	Fat	Calories	Carbs	Protein
TOTALS					
Satisfied after eating?					

Meal 5	Portion Sizes	Fat	Calories	Carbs	Protein
TOTALS					
Satisfied after eating?					

DAY #:___________

Meal 1	Portion Sizes	Fat	Calories	Carbs	Protein
TOTALS					
Satisfied after eating?					

Meal 2	Portion Sizes	Fat	Calories	Carbs	Protein
TOTALS					
Satisfied after eating?					

Notes

Meal 3	Portion Sizes	Fat	Calories	Carbs	Protein
TOTALS					
Satisfied after eating?					

Meal 4	Portion Sizes	Fat	Calories	Carbs	Protein
TOTALS					
Satisfied after eating?					

Meal 5	Portion Sizes	Fat	Calories	Carbs	Protein
TOTALS					
Satisfied after eating?					

DAY #:____________

Meal 1	Portion Sizes	Fat	Calories	Carbs	Protein
TOTALS					
Satisfied after eating?					

Meal 2	Portion Sizes	Fat	Calories	Carbs	Protein
TOTALS					
Satisfied after eating?					

Notes

Meal 3	Portion Sizes		Fat	Calories	Carbs	Protein
TOTALS						
Satisfied after eating?						

Meal 4	Portion Sizes		Fat	Calories	Carbs	Protein
TOTALS						
Satisfied after eating?						

Meal 5	Portion Sizes		Fat	Calories	Carbs	Protein
TOTALS						
Satisfied after eating?						

DAY #:___________

Meal 1	Portion Sizes	Fat	Calories	Carbs	Protein
TOTALS					
Satisfied after eating?					

Meal 2	Portion Sizes	Fat	Calories	Carbs	Protein
TOTALS					
Satisfied after eating?					

Notes

Meal 3	Portion Sizes	Fat	Calories	Carbs	Protein
TOTALS					
Satisfied after eating?					

Meal 4	Portion Sizes	Fat	Calories	Carbs	Protein
TOTALS					
Satisfied after eating?					

Meal 5	Portion Sizes	Fat	Calories	Carbs	Protein
TOTALS					
Satisfied after eating?					

DAY #:__________

Meal 1	Portion Sizes	Fat	Calories	Carbs	Protein
TOTALS					
Satisfied after eating?					

Meal 2	Portion Sizes	Fat	Calories	Carbs	Protein
TOTALS					
Satisfied after eating?					

Notes

Meal 3	Portion Sizes	Fat	Calories	Carbs	Protein
TOTALS					
Satisfied after eating?					

Meal 4	Portion Sizes	Fat	Calories	Carbs	Protein
TOTALS					
Satisfied after eating?					

Meal 5	Portion Sizes	Fat	Calories	Carbs	Protein
TOTALS					
Satisfied after eating?					

DAY #:___________

Meal 1	Portion Sizes	Fat	Calories	Carbs	Protein
TOTALS					
Satisfied after eating?					

Meal 2	Portion Sizes	Fat	Calories	Carbs	Protein
TOTALS					
Satisfied after eating?					

Notes

Meal 3	Portion Sizes	Fat	Calories	Carbs	Protein
TOTALS					
Satisfied after eating?					

Meal 4	Portion Sizes	Fat	Calories	Carbs	Protein
TOTALS					
Satisfied after eating?					

Meal 5	Portion Sizes	Fat	Calories	Carbs	Protein
TOTALS					
Satisfied after eating?					

DAY #: ___________

Meal 1	Portion Sizes	Fat	Calories	Carbs	Protein
TOTALS					
Satisfied after eating?					

Meal 2	Portion Sizes	Fat	Calories	Carbs	Protein
TOTALS					
Satisfied after eating?					

Notes

Meal 3	Portion Sizes	Fat	Calories	Carbs	Protein
TOTALS					
Satisfied after eating?					

Meal 4	Portion Sizes	Fat	Calories	Carbs	Protein
TOTALS					
Satisfied after eating?					

Meal 5	Portion Sizes	Fat	Calories	Carbs	Protein
TOTALS					
Satisfied after eating?					

DAY #: ___________

Meal 1	Portion Sizes		Fat	Calories	Carbs	Protein
TOTALS						
Satisfied after eating?						

Meal 2	Portion Sizes		Fat	Calories	Carbs	Protein
TOTALS						
Satisfied after eating?						

Notes

Meal 3	Portion Sizes	Fat	Calories	Carbs	Protein
TOTALS					
Satisfied after eating?					

Meal 4	Portion Sizes	Fat	Calories	Carbs	Protein
TOTALS					
Satisfied after eating?					

Meal 5	Portion Sizes	Fat	Calories	Carbs	Protein
TOTALS					
Satisfied after eating?					

DAY #:____________

Meal 1	Portion Sizes	Fat	Calories	Carbs	Protein
TOTALS					
Satisfied after eating?					

Meal 2	Portion Sizes	Fat	Calories	Carbs	Protein
TOTALS					
Satisfied after eating?					

Notes

Meal 3	Portion Sizes	Fat	Calories	Carbs	Protein
TOTALS					
Satisfied after eating?					

Meal 4	Portion Sizes	Fat	Calories	Carbs	Protein
TOTALS					
Satisfied after eating?					

Meal 5	Portion Sizes	Fat	Calories	Carbs	Protein
TOTALS					
Satisfied after eating?					

DAY #:____________

Meal 1	Portion Sizes		Fat	Calories	Carbs	Protein
TOTALS						
Satisfied after eating?						

Meal 2	Portion Sizes		Fat	Calories	Carbs	Protein
TOTALS						
Satisfied after eating?						

Notes

Meal 3	Portion Sizes	Fat	Calories	Carbs	Protein
TOTALS					
Satisfied after eating?					

Meal 4	Portion Sizes	Fat	Calories	Carbs	Protein
TOTALS					
Satisfied after eating?					

Meal 5	Portion Sizes	Fat	Calories	Carbs	Protein
TOTALS					
Satisfied after eating?					

DAY #:___________

Meal 1	Portion Sizes		Fat	Calories	Carbs	Protein
TOTALS						
Satisfied after eating?						

Meal 2	Portion Sizes		Fat	Calories	Carbs	Protein
TOTALS						
Satisfied after eating?						

Notes

Meal 3	Portion Sizes	Fat	Calories	Carbs	Protein
TOTALS					
Satisfied after eating?					

Meal 4	Portion Sizes	Fat	Calories	Carbs	Protein
TOTALS					
Satisfied after eating?					

Meal 5	Portion Sizes	Fat	Calories	Carbs	Protein
TOTALS					
Satisfied after eating?					

DAY #:____________

Meal 1	Portion Sizes		Fat	Calories	Carbs	Protein
TOTALS						
Satisfied after eating?						

Meal 2	Portion Sizes		Fat	Calories	Carbs	Protein
TOTALS						
Satisfied after eating?						

Notes

Meal 3	Portion Sizes		Fat	Calories	Carbs	Protein
TOTALS						
Satisfied after eating?						

Meal 4	Portion Sizes		Fat	Calories	Carbs	Protein
TOTALS						
Satisfied after eating?						

Meal 5	Portion Sizes		Fat	Calories	Carbs	Protein
TOTALS						
Satisfied after eating?						

www.ingramcontent.com/pod-product-compliance
Lightning Source LLC
Chambersburg PA
CBHW080246290526
45790CB00005B/1723

* 9 7 8 1 5 1 1 4 2 0 7 1 6 *